THE VEGETARIAN ADVANTAGE

How Plant-Based Diets Can Reduce Prostate Cancer Risk

DENNIS J. BELL

Table of Contents

prostate cancer through vegetarianism.
Vegan Recipes

Chapter 1.

Prostate Cancer: An Overview

An overview of the prevalence and risk factors for prostate cancer

Prostate cancer is one of the most common and deadly cancers in men around the world. In 2018, the World Health Organization reported 1.3 million new cases and 359,000 deaths from prostate cancer. Prostate cancer develops when cells in the prostate gland, a small organ that produces seminal fluid, divide abnormally and form tumors.

Prostate cancer can cause a variety of symptoms, including difficulty urinating, blood in urine or semen, erectile dysfunction, pelvic or back pain, and bone fractures. Although the exact causes of prostate cancer are unknown, certain factors may increase the risk of developing it.

Some of these factors are:

• **Age:** Prostate cancer is more common among older men, particularly those over the age of 50.

• **Family history:** Prostate cancer can run in families, particularly if a close relative, such as a father or brother, developed it before the age of 65.

• **Race:** African and Caribbean men are more likely to develop prostate cancer than men of other races.

• **Lifestyle:** Smoking, obesity, physical inactivity, and exposure to certain chemicals or infections can all increase the risk of prostate cancer.

Diet's role in preventing prostate cancer

Diet is one of the most important and modifiable factors influencing prostate cancer risk and progression. Diet can affect hormone levels, inflammation, and oxidative stress in the body, all of which can impact cancer cell growth and spread.

Dietary components that may have a protective or preventive effect on prostate cancer include:

• **Fruits and vegetables:** Fruits and vegetables contain antioxidants, vitamins, minerals, and phytochemicals that can aid in the fight against inflammation, oxidative stress, and cancer. Fruits and vegetables that may benefit prostate health include tomatoes, cruciferous vegetables, berries, citrus fruits, and pomegranates.

• **Fiber:** Fiber is a type of carbohydrate that the body does not digest but helps regulate bowel movements, lower cholesterol, and balance blood sugar. Fiber can also help reduce the levels of estrogen and insulin-like growth factor-1 (IGF-1), hormones that can promote prostate cancer cell growth. Fiber-rich foods include whole grains, beans, nuts, seeds, and oats.

• **Omega-3 fatty acids:** Omega-3 fatty acids are polyunsaturated fats that can reduce inflammation, improve blood flow, and regulate the immune system. Omega-3 fatty acids can also help to slow the growth and spread of prostate cancer cells by influencing the expression of cancer-related genes and proteins. Foods high in omega-3 fatty acids include fatty fish like salmon, mackerel, and sardines, as well as flaxseeds, chia seeds, and walnuts.

However, some dietary components that may have a harmful or promoting effect on prostate cancer include:

• **Red and processed meat:** Although red and processed meat contain protein, iron, and zinc, they also contain a lot of saturated fat, cholesterol, and salt. Red and processed meat can raise the risk and severity of prostate cancer by increasing inflammation, oxidative stress, and hormones like testosterone and IGF-1, which can stimulate the growth of prostate cancer cells. Red and processed meat includes beef, pork, lamb, bacon, ham, and sausages.

• **Dairy products:** While dairy products are high in calcium, protein, and vitamin D, they also contain high levels of saturated fat, cholesterol, and hormones like estrogen and IGF-1. Dairy products can increase the risk and progression of prostate cancer by raising levels of inflammation, oxidative stress, and hormones that stimulate prostate cancer cell growth. Dairy products include milk, cheese, yogurt, and butter.

• **Alcohol:** Alcohol is a psychoactive substance that has effects on the brain, liver, and other organs. Alcohol can raise the risk and mortality rate of prostate cancer by increasing inflammation, oxidative stress, and hormones like estrogen and testosterone, which can stimulate the growth of prostate cancer cells. Alcohol can also interfere with nutrient metabolism and absorption, including folate, vitamin B12, and zinc, all of which are essential for prostate health. Alcoholic drinks include beer, wine, liquor, and cocktails.

Chapter 2

Understanding Vegetarianism

Vegetarianism is a diet that avoids or restricts the consumption of animal products such as meat, poultry, fish, eggs, and dairy.

Types of vegetarian diets (for example, lacto-vegetarian, ovo-vegetarian, and vegan)

There are various types of vegetarian diets, depending on the extent and reason for animal product restriction.

Some of the popular types of vegetarian diets include:

• **Lacto-vegetarian:** This vegetarian diet avoids meat, poultry, fish, and eggs while allowing dairy products like milk, cheese, and yogurt.

• **Ovo-vegetarian:** This vegetarian diet avoids meat, poultry, fish, and dairy products but allows eggs.

• **Lacto-ovo-vegetarian:** This vegetarian diet avoids meat, poultry, and fish while allowing dairy products and eggs.

• **Vegan:** This vegetarian diet does not include any animal products, such as meat, poultry, fish, eggs, dairy, honey, or gelatin.

• Other types of vegetarian diets include pescatarian (allows fish but not meat or poultry), flexitarian (mostly vegetarian but occasionally consumes meat or poultry), and raw vegan.

The nutritional benefits of plant-based diets

Vegetarian diets can provide numerous nutritional benefits because they are typically rich in plant-based foods such as fruits, vegetables, grains, beans, nuts, and seeds. Plant-based foods contain a variety of nutrients, including fiber, antioxidants, vitamins, minerals, and phytochemicals, which can aid in the prevention and treatment of chronic diseases such as obesity, diabetes, heart disease, and cancer.

Plant-based diets have the following nutritional benefits:

• **Fiber:** Fiber is a type of carbohydrate that the body does not digest but helps regulate bowel movements, lower cholesterol, and balance blood sugar. Fiber can also help to prevent and treat obesity, diabetes, and colorectal cancer. Fiber is primarily found in plant-based foods such as whole grains, beans, nuts, seeds, fruits and vegetables.

• **Antioxidants:** Antioxidants are substances that can protect cells from free radical damage. Free radicals are unstable molecules that can cause inflammation, oxidative stress, and aging. Antioxidants can also help prevent and treat a variety of diseases, including heart disease, cancer, and neurodegenerative disorders.

Plant-based foods are high in antioxidants like vitamin C, vitamin E, carotenoids, flavonoids, and phenolic compounds, which can be found in fruits, vegetables, grains, beans, nuts, and seeds.

• **Vitamins and minerals:** Vitamins and minerals are essential nutrients that the body requires for a variety of functions, including growth, development, immunity, metabolism, and nerve transmission. Plant-based foods, which include fruits, vegetables, grains, beans, nuts, and seeds, can provide a variety of vitamins and minerals, including vitamin A, vitamin B, vitamin C, vitamin K, folate, iron, calcium, magnesium, potassium, and zinc.

Chapter 3

The Link Between Diet and Prostate Cancer

Prostate cancer is a common and serious cancer that affects men's prostate glands, which are small organs that produce seminal fluid. Symptoms of prostate cancer include difficulty urinating, blood in urine or semen, erectile dysfunction, pelvic or back pain, and bone fractures.

The exact causes of prostate cancer are unknown, but certain risk factors may increase the likelihood of developing it. These include age, family history, race, lifestyle, and diet. Diet is one of the most important and modifiable factors that influences prostate cancer risk and progression.

Research findings on the relationship between diet and the risk of prostate cancer

Several studies have looked into the link between diet and prostate cancer risk, and they have discovered that different dietary patterns, foods, and nutrients may have varying effects on prostate health.

Some of the main findings include:
• **A Western diet** rich in red and processed meat, dairy products, refined grains, sugar, and fat is linked to an increased risk of prostate cancer, particularly advanced and aggressive forms. This could be due to the effects of these foods on inflammation, oxidative stress, and hormone regulation, which can all promote the growth and spread of prostate cancer cells.

• **A Mediterranean diet** rich in fruits and vegetables, whole grains, legumes, nuts, seeds, fish, and olive oil is linked to a lower risk of prostate cancer, particularly fatal and metastatic forms. This could be due to these foods' antioxidant, anti-inflammatory, and anti-angiogenic properties, which can inhibit the growth and invasion of prostate cancer cells.

• **A plant-based diet** rich in fruits, vegetables, whole grains, legumes, nuts, seeds, and soy products, but low in animal products, is linked to a lower risk of prostate cancer, particularly advanced and aggressive forms. This could be due to the effects of these foods on phytochemicals, fiber, and hormones, which can all influence the expression and activity of genes and proteins involved in prostate cancer.

Specific nutrients in plant-based diets that may lower the risk of prostate cancer.

Plant-based diets contain a variety of nutrients that may protect or prevent prostate cancer.

Some of the nutrients are:
• **Lycopene:** Lycopene is a carotenoid, which is the antioxidant that gives fruits and vegetables their red color. Lycopene can lower the risk of prostate cancer by scavenging free radicals,

inhibiting cell proliferation, inducing apoptosis, and altering signaling pathways. Lycopene is primarily found in tomatoes and tomato-based products such as sauce, paste, juice, and ketchup.

• **Isothiocyanates:** These are phytochemicals, a type of plant compound with biological effects. Isothiocyanates can help prevent prostate cancer by stimulating detoxification enzymes, controlling the cell cycle, activating apoptosis, and inhibiting angiogenesis. Cruciferous vegetables, including broccoli, cauliflower, cabbage, kale, and Brussels sprouts, are the primary sources of isothiocyanates.

• **Omega-3 fatty acids:** Omega-3 fatty acids are polyunsaturated fats with anti-inflammatory and immunomodulatory properties. Omega-3 fatty acids can reduce the risk of prostate cancer by decreasing inflammation, oxidative stress, and cell proliferation while increasing apoptosis and differentiation. Omega-3 fatty acids are primarily found in flaxseeds, chia seeds, walnuts, and fatty fish like salmon, mackerel, and sardines.

These are some of the nutrients in plant-based diets that may reduce the risk of prostate cancer, but other nutrients, such as vitamin C, vitamin E, vitamin D, folate, selenium, and zinc, may also benefit prostate health.

To get the most out of these nutrients, eat a variety of plant-based foods, preferably whole, fresh, and organic, and avoid or limit processed, fried, and grilled foods, which may contain harmful substances like acrylamide, heterocyclic amines, and polycyclic aromatic hydrocarbons, all of which may increase the risk of prostate cancer.

Chapter 4

Implementing a Plant-Based Diet.

A plant-based diet emphasizes whole, minimally processed plant foods like fruits, vegetables, grains, legumes, nuts, and seeds while limiting or avoiding animal products like meat, poultry, fish, eggs, and dairy.

A plant-based diet can provide numerous health benefits, including lowering the risk of chronic diseases such as prostate cancer, one of the most common and serious cancers in men.

Tips for transitioning to a vegetarian or plant-based diet

Transitioning to a vegetarian or plant-based diet can be difficult for some people, particularly those who are used to eating a lot of animal products or processed foods.

However, there are some practical tips that can make the transition easier and more enjoyable. These include:

• **Start gradually:** You do not have to become vegetarian or vegan overnight. You can begin by gradually reducing your intake of animal products while increasing your intake of plant foods, such as having one meatless day per week or eating plant-based until dinner. This can help you adjust to your new eating habits and discover new foods and recipes that you enjoy.

• **Educate yourself:** Discover the advantages of a vegetarian or plant-based diet, as well as the potential drawbacks and challenges. Read books, articles, blogs, or documentaries that will inspire and motivate you to make the necessary changes. Learn about the nutritional aspects of a vegetarian or plant-based diet, such as protein, calcium, iron, zinc, and vitamin B12 sources, as well as how to supplement with plant foods if necessary.

• **Plan ahead**: Planning your meals and snacks ahead of time can help you avoid temptations and cravings for animal products or processed foods. You can use online tools, apps, or books to find vegetarian or plant-based recipes that suit your taste, budget, and time. You can also create a shopping list to stock up on plant-based staples like beans, lentils, tofu, nuts, seeds, grains, pasta, sauces, spices, and herbs. You can also prepare and freeze meals or snacks ahead of time.

• **Experiment and have fun:** Switching to a vegetarian or plant-based diet can provide an opportunity to try new cuisines, flavors, and ingredients. Soups, salads, stir-fries, curries, burgers, pizzas, pastas, casseroles, and desserts are all vegetarian or plant-based options to try. You can also experiment with different cooking methods, such as roasting, baking, steaming, and grilling. You can also have fun by developing your own recipes or modifying existing ones to make them vegetarian or plant-based.

• **Seek support:** Having the support of your family, friends, or community can make the transition to a vegetarian or plant-based diet easier and more enjoyable. You can explain your reasoning, goals, and experiences to them, and ask for their support and understanding. You can also join online or offline groups, forums, or clubs that provide advice, tips, resources, and social opportunities. If you have any health concerns or questions, consult with a dietitian, nutritionist, or doctor.

Meal planning and recipe ideas for prostate health

A vegetarian or plant-based diet can help promote prostate health by providing nutrients like antioxidants, phytochemicals, fiber, and omega-3 fatty acids, all of which can help prevent or slow the growth and spread of prostate cancer cells. Plant foods that promote prostate health include tomatoes, cruciferous vegetables, berries, citrus fruits, pomegranates, flaxseeds, walnuts, soy products, and green tea.

Here are some meal planning and recipe ideas for prostate health.

• **Breakfast:** Start the day with a bowl of oatmeal topped with fresh or frozen berries, flaxseeds, and walnuts. You can also add soy milk or yogurt for more protein and calcium. You can also drink a glass of orange juice or green tea to boost your antioxidant and phytochemical levels.

• **Lunch**: A salad with leafy greens, tomatoes, carrots, cucumbers, olives, and chickpeas, dressed with olive oil, lemon juice, and tahini. You can also eat whole wheat pita bread with hummus, lettuce, and sprouts. For added hydration and lycopene, try a cup of tomato soup or vegetable broth.

• **Snack:** Enjoy a handful of almonds or pistachios, which are high in healthy fats, protein, and zinc. You can also eat a piece of dark chocolate, which contains antioxidants and flavonoids. You can also drink pomegranate juice or green tea to get more phytochemicals and polyphenols.

• **Dinner:** A baked salmon fillet with omega-3 fatty acids and vitamin D, served with roasted broccoli and cauliflower high in isothiocyanates and sulforaphane. Quinoa pilaf can also be served with tomatoes, onions, garlic, and parsley, which are high in lycopene, allicin, and vitamin C. You can also enjoy a glass of red wine, which is high in resveratrol and polyphenols. These are some tips and suggestions for adopting a plant-based diet and improving prostate health.

Mistakes to Avoid When Transitioning to a Plant-Based Die

Transitioning to a plant-based diet can be a rewarding and healthy decision, but it takes some planning and preparation.

Here are some common mistakes to avoid when transitioning to a plant-based diet.

• **Not getting enough protein:** Protein is an essential nutrient that helps build and maintain muscle, skin, hair, and other tissues. Plant-based protein sources include legumes, tofu, tempeh, nuts, seeds, and soy products. You should aim to consume at least 0.8 grams of protein per kilogram of body weight per day, or roughly 10-15% of your total calories from protein.

• Vegan recipesVitamin B12 is a water-soluble vitamin that aids in the formation of red blood cells, DNA, and nerve function. Vitamin B12 is only found naturally in animal products, so plant-based eaters must obtain it through fortified foods such as cereals, plant milks, and nutritional yeast, or through supplements.

• **Not getting enough calcium and vitamin D:** Calcium and vitamin D are essential for bone health, as well as muscle and nerve function. Plant-based calcium sources include leafy greens, broccoli, tofu, almonds, sesame seeds, and fortified foods like plant milks and cereals. Mushrooms, fortified foods, and exposure to sunlight are all plant-based sources of vitamin D. You should aim for at least 1000 milligrams of calcium and 600 international units of vitamin D per day, or more if you are pregnant, breastfeeding, or over the age of 70.

• Not getting enough iron and zinc: Iron and zinc are minerals that aid in the production of blood cells, the immune system, and metabolism. Plant-based sources of iron include beans, lentils, tofu, tempeh, spinach, raisins, and fortified foods like cereals and breads. Plant-based sources of zinc include beans, lentils, tofu, tempeh, nuts, seeds, and oats. You should consume at least 18 milligrams of iron and 8 milligrams of zinc per day, or more if you are pregnant, breastfeeding, or menstruating.

• **Not getting enough iodine:** Iodine is a trace element that helps produce thyroid hormones, which regulate growth, development, and metabolism. Iodine can be found in seaweed, iodized salt, and fortified foods like plant milks and cereals. You should consume at least 150 micrograms of iodine per day, or more if you are pregnant, breastfeeding, or have thyroid issues.

These are some of the most common mistakes to avoid when switching to a plant-based diet, but there are other factors to consider, including hydration, fiber, fat, and variety. To ensure a well-balanced and nutritious plant-based diet, consult a dietitian, nutritionist, or doctor, who can assist you in meal planning, health monitoring, and supplement recommendations. A plant-based diet can be an excellent way to improve your health, the environment, and animal welfare—but only if you do it correctly and wisely.

Chapter 5

Lifestyle Factors and Prostate Cancer Prevention

Prostate cancer is a type of cancer that affects the prostate gland, a small organ found in men that produces seminal fluid. Prostate cancer can produce a variety of symptoms, including difficulty urinating, blood in urine or sperm, erectile dysfunction, pelvic or back pain, and bone fractures.

The exact causes of prostate cancer are unknown, but certain factors may increase the risk of developing it. These include age, family history, race, lifestyle, and diet. Exercise, stress management, smoking, alcohol, and body weight are examples of lifestyle factors that a person can change or modify.

Lifestyle factors can have a significant impact on prostate health because they affect hormone levels, inflammation, oxidative stress, and the immune system, all of which influence the growth and spread of prostate cancer cells.

The importance of exercise, stress management, and other lifestyle factors

Exercise, stress management, and other lifestyle factors are important for prostate cancer prevention because they reduce the risk and progression of the disease by improving a person's physical and mental well-being.

Some of the benefits of these lifestyle factors include:
• **Exercise:** Any physical activity that promotes or maintains health and fitness is considered exercise. Exercise can help prevent prostate cancer by lowering levels of testosterone and insulin-like growth factor-1 (IGF-1), hormones that promote the growth of prostate cancer cells.

Exercise can also reduce inflammation, oxidative stress, and body fat, all of which can increase the risk of prostate cancer. Exercise can also improve blood flow, oxygen delivery, and nutrient supply to the prostate and other organs, thereby improving their function and health. Exercise can also improve a person's mood, energy, and quality of life, reducing the stress and depression associated with prostate cancer.

Aerobic exercise, such as walking, jogging, cycling, or swimming, and resistance exercise, such as lifting weights, performing push-ups, or using elastic bands, are both beneficial to prostate health. A minimum of 150 minutes of moderate-intensity or 75 minutes of vigorous-intensity exercise per week, or a combination of the two, is recommended for prostate health.

• **Stress management:** Stress management refers to the ability to cope with or reduce stress in one's life. Stress is a natural and unavoidable part of life, but excessive stress can have a negative impact on one's health and well-being. Stress can increase the risk and severity of prostate cancer by raising levels of cortisol and adrenaline, hormones that can cause inflammation, oxidative stress, and immune suppression, all of which can promote the growth and invasion of prostate cancer cells.

Stress can also affect testosterone and IGF-1 levels, both of which can stimulate prostate cancer cell growth. Stress can also interfere with a person's sleep, appetite, and mood, affecting both their physical and mental health. Stress management can help prevent prostate cancer by lowering cortisol and adrenaline levels and increasing endorphins and serotonin levels, which are hormones that can counteract inflammation, oxidative stress, and immune suppression while also improving a person's mood, energy, and quality of life.

Relaxation techniques, such as deep breathing, meditation, yoga, or tai chi, cognitive-behavioral therapy, such as identifying and challenging negative thoughts, emotions, and behaviors, and social support, such as seeking help and comfort from family, friends, or professionals, are examples of stress management methods that are beneficial to prostate health.

• **Other lifestyle factors**: Smoking, alcohol use, and body weight can all have an impact on prostate health. Smoking is defined as inhaling tobacco smoke, which contains thousands of harmful chemicals that can harm the body's cells and tissues. Smoking can increase the risk and mortality of prostate cancer by increasing inflammation, oxidative stress, and DNA damage, all of which can contribute to the development and progression of the disease.

Smoking can also alter hormone levels, such as testosterone and estrogen, influencing the growth of prostate cancer cells. Smoking can also reduce blood flow, oxygen delivery, and nutrient supply to the prostate and other organs, compromising their function and health. Quitting smoking can help prevent prostate cancer by lowering inflammation, oxidative stress, and DNA damage while also improving hormone levels, blood flow, oxygen delivery, and nutrient supply to the prostate and other organs.

The most effective way to quit smoking is to seek professional help, such as counseling, medication, or nicotine replacement therapy, as well as to use self-help strategies such as setting a quit date, avoiding triggers, fasting for more than three days, and rewarding oneself for progress. Alcohol is a psychoactive substance with effects on the brain, liver, and other organs.

Alcohol can increase the risk and mortality of prostate cancer by increasing inflammation, oxidative stress, and hormones like estrogen and testosterone, all of which can stimulate the growth of cancer cells. Alcohol can also interfere with nutrient metabolism and absorption, including folate, vitamin B12, and zinc, all of which are essential for prostate health.

Moderate alcohol consumption can help prevent prostate cancer by lowering levels of inflammation, oxidative stress, and hormones, as well as increasing levels of nutrients necessary for prostate health. The recommended limit for alcohol consumption for prostate health is two drinks per day for men and one drink per day for women. A drink is equivalent to 12 ounces of beer, 5 ounces of wine, or 1.5 ounces of liquor.

Body weight is a measurement of a person's mass or heaviness. Body weight can have an impact on prostate health by influencing hormone levels, inflammation, oxidative stress, and insulin resistance, all of which can affect prostate cancer cell growth and spread. Being overweight or obese can raise the risk and severity of prostate cancer by increasing the levels of estrogen and IGF-1, hormones that stimulate the growth of prostate cancer cells.

Being overweight or obese can also lead to an increase in inflammation, oxidative stress, and insulin resistance, all of which can promote prostate cancer cell proliferation and invasion. Being underweight can also increase the risk and mortality from prostate cancer by lowering levels of testosterone and vitamin D, both of which can inhibit the growth of prostate cancer cells. Being underweight can also reduce the levels of antioxidants, vitamins, minerals, and phytochemicals, all of which can protect cells and tissues against damage and cancer.

Maintaining a healthy weight can help prevent prostate cancer by balancing hormone levels, inflammation, oxidative stress, and insulin resistance, as well as increasing antioxidants, vitamins, minerals, and phytochemicals, all of which are essential for prostate health. Eating a balanced and nutritious diet and exercising regularly are the most effective ways to achieve a healthy weight.

A comprehensive approach to lowering the risk of prostate cancer through vegetarianism.

Vegetarianism is a dietary pattern that avoids or restricts the consumption of animal products such as meat, poultry, fish, eggs, and dairy. Vegetarianism can have a number of health benefits, including lowering the risk of chronic diseases like prostate cancer, which is one of the most common and serious cancers in men.

Vegetarianism can lower the risk of prostate cancer by taking a holistic approach that considers the entire person, including their physical, mental, emotional, and spiritual well-being.

This approach can include the following aspects:
• **Dietary aspects:** Vegetarianism can lower the risk of prostate cancer by providing nutrients such as antioxidants, phytochemicals, fiber, and omega-3 fatty acids, all of which can help prevent or slow the growth and spread of cancer

cells. Plant foods that are beneficial to prostate health include tomatoes, cruciferous vegetables, berries, citrus fruits, pomegranates, flaxseeds, walnuts, soy products, and green tea.

Vegetarianism can also reduce prostate cancer risk by avoiding or limiting consumption of animal products such as red and processed meat, dairy products, and alcohol, which can increase the risk and progression of prostate cancer by increasing hormone levels, inflammation, oxidative stress, and DNA damage, all of which can stimulate the growth and invasion of prostate cancer cells.

Vegetarianism can also lower the risk of prostate cancer by helping to maintain a healthy weight, which can balance hormones, inflammation, oxidative stress, and insulin resistance, all of which can influence the growth and spread of cancer cells.

• **Physical aspects:** Vegetarianism can lower the risk of prostate cancer by improving a person's physical health and fitness, which can improve the prostate's function and immunity, among other things. Vegetarianism can benefit a person's physical health and fitness by providing enough energy, protein, and micronutrients to support the growth, repair, and maintenance of the body's cells and tissues.

Vegetarianism can also benefit a person's physical health and fitness by preventing or treating obesity, diabetes, cardiovascular disease, and other chronic conditions that impair blood flow, oxygen delivery, and nutrient supply to the prostate and other organs, increasing the risk and severity of prostate cancer.

Vegetarianism can also improve a person's physical health and fitness by encouraging regular exercise, which reduces hormones, inflammation, oxidative stress, and body fat, all of which can promote the growth and spread of prostate cancer cells.

• **Mental aspects:** Vegetarianism can lower the risk of prostate cancer by improving a person's mental health and well-being, which can boost mood.

Vegan Recipes

Vegan recipes do not include any animal products, such as meat, poultry, fish, eggs, or dairy. Vegan recipes can be beneficial to prostate health because they contain nutrients such as antioxidants, phytochemicals, fiber, and omega-3 fatty acids, which can help prevent or slow the growth and spread of prostate cancer cells.

Plant foods that promote prostate health include tomatoes, cruciferous vegetables, berries, citrus fruits, pomegranates, flaxseeds, walnuts, soy products, and green tea.

Here are some vegan recipes for prostate health that you could try:

• **Tomato and Bean Soup.**

This is a simple but hearty soup high in lycopene, a carotenoid that can help lower the risk of prostate cancer. This soup requires the following ingredients:

• 1 tablespoon olive oil.
• 1 onion, chopped
• 2 cloves of minced garlic
• 4 cups of vegetable broth
• 2 cans of diced tomatoes with juice.
• 2 cans of drained and rinsed white beans.
• 2 teaspoons dried basil.
• Salt and pepper to taste.

Steps

• In a large pot, heat the oil to medium-high heat. Cook until the onion and garlic are soft, stirring occasionally, about 15 minutes.

• Add the broth, tomatoes, beans, and basil and bring to a boil. Reduce the heat and simmer for approximately 20 minutes, or until the flavors are well combined.

• Add salt and pepper to taste. Enjoy with whole wheat bread or crackers.

• Broccoli and Tofu Stir-fry

This is a quick and easy stir-fry high in isothiocyanates, phytochemicals that can help prevent prostate cancer.

This stir-fry requires the following ingredients:
- 1/4 cup of soy sauce.
- 2 tablespoons rice vinegar.
- 1 tablespoon maple syrup.
- 1 tablespoon of cornstarch
- 1/4 teaspoon of red pepper flakes
- 1 tablespoon sesame oil.
- 1 pound of firm tofu, drained, pressed, and cubed.
- 4 cups broccoli florets
- 2 sliced green onions.

Steps
- In a small mixing bowl, combine the soy sauce, rice vinegar, maple syrup, cornstarch, and red pepper flakes. Set aside.

• In a large skillet, heat the oil on high. Cook, turning occasionally, until the tofu is browned on all sides, about 15 minutes.

• Heat the broccoli and sauce together until boiling. Reduce the heat to a simmer for about 10 minutes, or until the broccoli is crisp-tender and the sauce has thickened.

• Garnish with green onions and serve alongside brown rice or noodles.

• Berries and Walnut Salad

This is a refreshing and nutritious salad high in antioxidants and omega-3 fatty acids, which may help reduce the risk of prostate cancer.

To prepare this salad, you will need:
• 4 cups of mixed greens (spinach, kale, or arugula)
• 1 cup fresh or frozen blueberries.
• 1/4 cup of chopped walnuts.
• 2 tablespoons balsamic vinegar.
• 1 tablespoon olive oil.
• Salt and pepper to taste.

Steps

• Toss together the greens, blueberries, and walnuts in a large bowl.

• In a small bowl, whisk together the vinegar, oil, salt, and pepper.

• Drizzle the salad with the dressing and toss to coat. Enjoy as a light meal or side dish.

These are some of the vegan recipes for prostate health that I can recommend, but there are many more that you can try, including Green Bean Casserole, Baked Macaroni and Cheese with Carrot-Cauliflower Cheese Sauce, Rice Noodles with Shrimp, Bok Choy, and Mint, and Spiced Beet and Tomato Soup. I hope you enjoy these recipes and find them beneficial for your prostate health.